Contents

Introduction

This book is a guide for individuals who are looking to improve their physical fitness and health in a short period of time. The book outlines a structured plan for a 30-day period with specific exercises and dietary recommendations that are designed to help the individual achieve their fitness goals.

By breaking down the process into manageable daily tasks, the book makes it easier for people to stick to their fitness goals and see progress over time. Additionally, the thirty-day format provides a sense of structure and accountability, as people can track their progress and see how far they have come by the end of the challenge. The book also includes tips, advice, and motivational messages to help people overcome obstacles and stay motivated throughout the thirty days. Overall, the goal of this thirty-day fitness challenge book is to help people develop a healthy and active lifestyle, and to feel proud of their accomplishments.

Chapter one

Fitness Challenge

Fitness Challenge is a program that encourages people to commit to exercising regularly. The idea is that by establishing a daily exercise habit, people can improve their physical fitness, feel better, and potentially make exercise a permanent part of their routine.

Importance of fitness challenge

The importance of the Fitness Challenge lies in its ability to help people form a habit. Habits are important because they allow us to perform tasks automatically, without having to think about them. By doing something every day for thirty days, it becomes easier for the brain to create a habit, and exercise can become a regular part of someone's daily routine.

A Fitness Challenge can also be a fun and social experience, as friends and family members can join in and support each other. This can increase accountability and help to keep participants on track, making it more likely that they will stick to the challenge and establish a habit.

Benefit of 30 days fitness challenge

Completing a 30-day fitness challenge can have several benefits, including:

1. Improved physical fitness: Regular exercise can help you become stronger, increase your endurance, and improve your overall physical health.

2. Better mental health: Exercise has been shown to reduce stress and anxiety and improve mood.

3. Increased energy levels: Regular physical activity can help increase your energy levels, making you feel more awake and alert.

4. Weight loss: Regular exercise combined with a healthy diet can help you lose weight and maintain a healthy body composition.

5. Improved sleep: Exercise has been shown to improve sleep quality, helping you fall asleep faster and sleep more deeply.

6. Increased confidence: Completing a fitness challenge can boost your self-confidence and self-esteem.

7. Improved habits: By committing to a fitness challenge, you are forming healthy habits that can last a lifetime.

8. Better heart health: Regular exercise can help lower blood pressure, improve circulation, and reduce the risk of heart disease.

Always listen to your body anytime you feel weak. Gradually increase the intensity and duration of your workout to avoid injury and ensure long-term success.

Chapter two

Pre-Challenge Preparation

Preparation is key to success when it comes to a fitness challenge. Whether you're a seasoned athlete or just starting out,

There are a few steps you can take to set yourself up for success and make the most of this opportunity.

1. Establish your goals: The first step to any fitness challenge is to figure out what you want to achieve.

2. Assess your current fitness level: Take stock of your current fitness level by trying out a variety of exercises and activities.

3. Create a workout plan: Once you have a good understanding of your goals and current fitness level, it's time to create a workout plan.

4. Find a workout buddy: Having a workout partner can be a great way to stay motivated and accountable.

5. Stock up on supplies: Make sure you have all the equipment and supplies you need to complete your workouts, including

comfortable clothing and sneakers, water bottles, towels, and any other gear that will help you stay comfortable and focused.

6. Plan your meals: Eating a nutritious, balanced diet is key to supporting your fitness goals. Plan your meals ahead of time and make sure you have plenty of healthy options on hand, such as fresh fruits and vegetables, lean protein, and whole grains.

7. Stay hydrated: Proper hydration is essential to your overall health and fitness, so make sure you are drinking plenty of water throughout the day.

8. Track your progress: Keeping a record of your progress can be a great way to stay motivated and see the results of your efforts.

9. Be consistent: Consistency is key when it comes to a fitness challenge. Make a commitment to yourself to show up and do your best every day, even on days when you don't feel like it.

Remember, a thirty-day fitness challenge is not just about physical results, but also about developing healthy habits that will last a lifetime. By focusing on consistency, setting achievable goals, and taking care of yourself both physically and mentally, you'll be well on your way to success.

Chapter Three

Setting Realistic Goals

To achieve a visible result at the end of the program it is very important for you to set realistic goals and the goals include but not limited to. These are just the most important ones.

1. Determine your starting point: Before you can set a realistic goal, you need to know your starting point. This includes your current weight, body fat percentage, and overall fitness level. This information will help you determine how much progress you can realistically make in thirty days.

2. Identify your motivations: What is driving you to start this challenge? Whether it's to lose weight, build muscle, or improve your overall health, having a clear motivator will help you stay committed to your goal.

3. Consider your schedule: Evaluate your schedule and determine how much time you can realistically dedicate to your fitness challenge each day. This will help you set achievable goals and avoid burnout.

4. Set realistic weight loss goals: A healthy rate of weight loss is 1-2 pounds per week. If you have more weight to lose, you may be able to lose more in the first few weeks, but it's essential to keep your goal realistic and sustainable. Losing more than 2 pounds per week can lead to muscle loss, which is not ideal.

5. Focus on progress, not perfection: The goal of a thirty-day fitness challenge is to make progress, not to be perfect. Try not to get discouraged if you happen to miss a session or treat yourself to something. Instead, concentrate on making steady progress and maintaining your dedication towards reaching your objectives.

6. Incorporate strength training: While cardio is an essential part of any fitness routine, incorporating strength training into your thirty-day fitness challenge will help you build muscle and improve your overall fitness. Focus on compound exercises that target multiple muscle groups at once, like squats and deadlifts.

7. Make healthy eating a priority: Diet is a crucial component of any fitness challenge, and making healthy eating choices is essential for success. Emphasize on consuming a nutritious diet consisting of a diversity of fruits, vegetables, proteins with low-fat content, and

nutritious fats. Minimize your consumption of foods that have undergone processing and excessive sugar.

With dedication and commitment, you can achieve your fitness goals and enjoy a healthier, happier life.

Chapter four

Choosing an Appropriate Workout Plan

The workout plan for the thirty-day fitness challenge is meant to increase your overall fitness level and improve your strength, endurance, and flexibility.

- Week 1: The first week will focus on building a foundation for the rest of the challenge. During this week, you will start with basic exercises that target different muscle groups and help you get used to a regular workout routine.

Day 1-3:

Warm-up: 5-minute brisk walk or jog

Exercise 1: Bodyweight squats (3 sets of 12 reps)

Exercise 2: Push-ups (3 sets of 12 reps)

Exercise 3: Plank (3 sets, hold for 30 seconds each)

Exercise 4: Lunges (3 sets of 12 reps on each leg)

Cool-down: 5-minute walk

Day 4-6:

Warm-up: 5-minute brisk walk or jog

Exercise 1: Dumbbell bicep curls (3 sets of 12 reps)

Exercise 2: Dumbbell triceps extensions (3 sets of 12 reps)

Exercise 3: Dumbbell hammer curls (3 sets of 12 reps)

Exercise 4: Dumbbell kickbacks (3 sets of 12 reps)

Cool-down: 5-minute walk

Day 7:

Rest day

- Week 2: During the second week, you will continue to build on the foundation you established during the first week and add some new exercises to your routine.

Day 8-10:

Warm-up: 5-minute brisk walk or jog

Exercise 1: Dumbbell squats (3 sets of 12 reps)

Exercise 2: Dumbbell chest press (3 sets of 12 reps)

Exercise 3: Dumbbell rows (3 sets of 12 reps)

Exercise 4: Dumbbell deadlifts (3 sets of 12 reps)

Cool-down: 5-minute walk

Day 11-13:

Warm-up: 5-minute brisk walk or jog

Exercise 1: Dumbbell lateral raises (3 sets of 12 reps)

Exercise 2: Dumbbell front raises (3 sets of 12 reps)

Exercise 3: Dumbbell overhead presses (3 sets of 12 reps)

Exercise 4: Dumbbell shrugs (3 sets of 12 reps)

Cool-down: 5-minute walk

Day 14:

Rest day

- Week 3: During the third week, you will continue to increase the intensity and complexity of your workout routine.

Day 15-17:

Warm-up: 5-minute brisk walk or jog

Exercise 1: Barbell squats (3 sets of 12 reps)

Exercise 2: Barbell bench press (3 sets of 12 reps)

Exercise 3: Barbell rows (3 sets of 12 reps)

Exercise 4: Barbell deadlifts (3 sets of 12 reps)

Cool-down: 5-minute walk

Day 18-20:

Warm-up: 5-minute brisk walk or jog

Exercise 1: Barbell bicep curls (3 sets of 12 reps)

Exercise 2: Barbell triceps extensions (3 sets of 12 reps)

Exercise 3: Barbell hammer curls (3 sets of 12 reps)

Exercise 4: Barbell kickbacks (3 sets of 12 reps)

Cool-down: 5-minute walk

Day 21:

Rest day

Day 22-24:

Warm-up: 5-minute brisk walk or jog

Exercise 1: Barbell squats (3 sets of 12 reps)

Exercise 2: Barbell deadlifts (3 sets of 12 reps)

Exercise 3: Barbell lunges (3 sets of 12 reps)

Exercise 4: Barbell calf raises (3 sets of 12 reps)

Cool-down: 5-minute walk

Day 25-27:

Warm-up: 5-minute brisk walk or jog

Exercise 1: Dumbbell chest press (3 sets of 12 reps)

Exercise 2: Dumbbell fly's (3 sets of 12 reps)

Exercise 3: Dumbbell pullovers (3 sets of 12 reps)

Exercise 4: Dumbbell pushups (3 sets of 12 reps)

Cool-down: 5-minute walk

Day 28-30:

Warm-up: 5-minute brisk walk or jog

Exercise 1: Barbell row (3 sets of 12 reps)

Exercise 2: Dumbbell bicep curls (3 sets of 12 reps)

Exercise 3: Dumbbell triceps extensions (3 sets of 12 reps)

Exercise 4: Dumbbell lateral raises (3 sets of 12 reps)

Cool-down: 5-minute walk

Remember to listen to your body and adjust the weights and reps accordingly. Don't push yourself too hard and give your body enough time to rest and recover between workouts.

Chapter five

Gathering Essential training equipment

For a thirty-day fitness challenge, you need to have the right equipment to maximize your results and stay safe while working out. Below is a list of essential items that you should consider investing in:

1. Exercise Mat: A high-quality exercise mat is a must-have for any workout routine. It will provide cushioning for your joints, making it easier and more comfortable to perform exercises such as push-ups, sit-ups, and yoga.

2. Resistance Bands: Resistance bands are a versatile piece of equipment that can be used to work out every muscle group in your body. They're also lightweight, making them easy to carry with you anywhere you go.

3. Dumbbells: Dumbbells are a classic piece of equipment that can be used for a variety of exercises. They come in different weights, so you can choose the ones that are best suited to your fitness level.

4. Kettlebells: Kettlebells are a great addition to your fitness equipment collection. They can be used for a variety of exercises, including swings, goblet squats, and Turkish get-ups.

5. Skipping Rope: Skipping is a great cardiovascular exercise that can be done anywhere. It's a fun and effective way to get your heart rate up and improve your endurance.

6. Foam Roller: A foam roller is a great tool for self-massage and recovery. It helps to loosen up tight muscles and can be especially helpful after a tough workout.

7. Yoga Block: Yoga blocks are an excellent tool for people of all levels, whether you're a beginner or an experienced yogi. They can be used to modify poses, making them more accessible, and they can also be used as a prop for balance and stability.

8. Heart Rate Monitor: Keeping track of your heart rate is an essential part of any fitness routine. A heart rate monitor will help you to stay within your target heart rate zone, ensuring that you're getting the most out of your workout.

9. Jump Rope: Jumping rope is a high-intensity cardio workout that can be done anywhere. It's a great way to improve your endurance and cardiovascular health…

10.	Stability ball: is a multi-functional exercise tool that can be utilized for an extensive range of workouts. It's great balance and strength, improving balance, and increasing core stability.

In conclusion, having the right equipment is essential for a successful fitness challenge. By investing in these items, you'll be able to maximize your results and stay safe while working out.

Chapter Six

Understanding the Importance of Nutrition

Nutrition plays a crucial role in a thirty-day fitness challenge and is often considered the backbone of a successful fitness program. Good nutrition provides the energy and nutrients required for the body to perform at its best during exercise, and it also supports recovery and muscle building. In this section of the book, we will discuss the importance of nutrition for a thirty-day fitness challenge and why it is crucial to pay attention to what you eat.

1. Adequate Fueling: Exercise demands energy, and the body obtains this energy from the food we eat.

2. Muscle Repair and Growth: After exercise, the body needs protein to repair and rebuild muscle tissue. Good sources of protein include chicken, fish, eggs, dairy products, beans, and nuts.

3. Recovery: Nutrition also plays a crucial role in recovery. After exercise, the body needs to replenish energy stores, repair muscle tissue, and reduce inflammation.

4. Weight Management: Nutrition is essential for weight management, and it is often the key to success in a thirty-day fitness challenge. By following a healthy diet, you can control.

5. Overall, Health: Good nutrition supports overall health and well-being, and it is essential for those participating in a thirty-day fitness challenge.

It is essential to pay attention to what you eat and make sure you are fueling your body with the energy and nutrients it needs to perform at its best. By incorporating a balanced diet with a variety of nutrient-dense foods, you can support your thirty-day fitness challenge and reach your goals.

Chapter seven

30 days fitness challenge

In these chapter the complete 30 days of the challenge would be discussed. Listed below are the lined-up plans.

Day 1-5: Warm-Up and Beginner Workouts

Welcome to your 30-Day Fitness Challenge! This challenge is designed to help you build a healthy and active lifestyle, no matter your current fitness level. The first five days of this challenge are dedicated to warming up and starting with beginner workouts.

Day 1: Warm-Up

Start your day by spending 5-10 minutes stretching and moving your body. This will help get your muscles ready for the workout ahead and prevent injury. Light cardio, such as jumping jacks or jogging in place, is also a good way to get your heart rate up and get your blood flowing.

Day 2: Bodyweight Squats

Bodyweight squats are a great way to work your legs and glutes. Start by positioning your feet hip-width apart, with your hands resting at your sides. Slowly bend your knees as if you're about to sit on a chair, making sure they don't extend beyond your toes. Rise back up to the starting position, keeping your weight balanced on your heels. Repeat this movement for 10-15 reps, working your way up to 3 sets as you progress through the challenge.

Day 3: Push-Ups

Push-ups are a classic exercise that works your chest, arms, and core. Start in a plank position, with your hands placed slightly wider than shoulder-width apart. Begin by bending down while maintaining a straight spine, then return to the starting position by pushing upward. Repeat this movement for 10-15 reps, working your way up to 3 sets as you progress through the challenge.

Day 4: Plank

The plank exercise is an excellent way to tone and strengthen your core muscles. Start in a push-up position, but instead of lowering yourself to the ground, hold the position with your arms straight and your back straight. Hold this position for 20-30 seconds and work your way up to a minute as you progress through the challenge.

Day 5: Lunges

Lunges provide an effective workout for your legs, glutes, and core muscles. Start with your feet hip-width apart and take a big step forward with one foot. Lower your body until both knees are bent at a 90-degree angle, and then push back up to the starting position. Repeat this movement for 10-15 reps on each leg, working your way up to 3 sets as you progress through the challenge.

These beginner workouts are designed to help you build a solid foundation for your fitness journey. As you progress through the challenge, you will add more exercises and increase the difficulty, but for now, focus on mastering these basics. Remember to warm up and cool down properly and listen to your body. If an exercise is too difficult, modify it or take a break. Your goal is to have fun and build a healthy and active lifestyle, not to push yourself too hard too fast.

So, get started with your first five days of the challenge, and remember to take it one day at a time. You've got this!

Day 6-10: Building Endurance and strength challenge.

Day 6 to 10 is the crucial period of a thirty-day fitness challenge as it is during this time that your body starts to adapt to the new routine and gets used to the increased physical activity. It is important to continue with your workout regimen and keep pushing yourself, while also paying attention to your body's needs. Here's what you can do to build endurance and strength during this period.

Day 6: On day six, focus on building your cardiovascular endurance. You can do this by engaging in high-intensity interval training (HIIT) or by going for a run. HIIT stands for High-Intensity Interval Training, which consists of repeating cycles of high-intensity exercise and recovery periods. For example, you can do 30 seconds of jumping jacks followed by 30 seconds of rest. Repeat this cycle for 10 minutes to get your heart rate up. If you prefer running, aim for a 30-minute run at a moderate pace.

Day 7: Take a break from your cardio routine and focus on strength training instead. You can do this by using resistance bands, weights, or your own body weight. Choose exercises that target multiple muscle groups, such as squats, lunges, push-ups, and pull-ups. Start with three sets of 10 reps for each exercise and gradually increase the number of sets and reps as you get stronger.

Day 8: Go back to your cardio routine, but this time, focus on building your endurance by going for a longer run or bike ride. Aim for at least 45 minutes of continuous activity at a moderate pace.

Day 9: It's important to take a day of rest after a challenging workout. Use this day to stretch and recover from the previous days' activities. Spend time stretching your muscles and foam rolling to help reduce muscle soreness.

Day 10: On day ten, challenge yourself to a more intense strength training workout. Focus on compound exercises that work multiple muscle groups at the same time, such as deadlifts, squats, and bench press. Start with three sets of 10 reps and gradually increase the weight as you get stronger.

Day 11-15: Increasing Intensity

Days 11-15 in a thirty-day fitness challenge can be seen as a gradual increase in intensity as the body adapts to the new physical demands. This stage of the challenge is important as it sets the foundation for the rest of the journey and prepares the body for the more challenging exercises ahead. The following are some suggestions for increasing intensity during this phase:

- Cardiovascular exercises: Incorporate more intense cardio exercises into your routine such as running, jumping jacks, high-intensity interval training (HIIT), and plyometric exercises. These exercises help to increase heart rate and burn more calories, leading to improved cardiovascular health.

- Strength training: Start incorporating strength training exercises into your routine such as push-ups, squats, lunges, and dumbbell exercises. These exercises help to build lean muscle mass and increase metabolism, leading to improved overall fitness and weight loss.

- Stretching: Make sure to include stretching exercises in your routine as they help to increase flexibility and prevent injury. Focus on stretching all major muscle groups, especially those that are most commonly tight such as the hips, hamstrings, and lower back.

- Variety: To avoid boredom and keep the body challenged, it is important to vary the types of exercises you perform. Try to incorporate different types of cardio and strength training exercises into your routine. This will also help to prevent plateaus and keep your progress moving forward.

- Challenge yourself: As you progress through the challenge, aim to increase the difficulty of your exercises. This can be done by increasing the number of repetitions, the weight of the resistance, or the length of the workout.

- Rest and recovery: It is important to listen to your body and allow it to rest and recover between workout sessions. This will help to prevent injury and improve overall performance.

Day 16-20: Mixing Up Workouts for Variety

Days 16-20 of a thirty-day fitness challenge should focus on mixing up workouts for variety. This can help prevent boredom and keep your body challenged, which can lead to better results. Here are a few workout ideas to try:

Day 16: Cardio Intervals

Start the day with a cardio workout that includes intervals. This means you'll alternate between high-intensity and low-intensity exercise for a set amount of time. For example, you could jog for 30 seconds and then walk for 30 seconds, repeating this pattern for 15 minutes.

Day 17: Strength Training

Strength training plays a crucial role in developing muscle mass and enhancing overall fitness levels. Focus on different muscle groups each day, such as arms and chest on Day 17. Use weights that challenge you but allow you to complete the recommended number of repetitions with proper form.

Day 18: Yoga

Yoga is a great workout for improving flexibility and reducing stress. There are many different types of yoga to choose from, so find one that you enjoy. A gentle, beginner-friendly yoga class would be a great way to stretch out your muscles and get in a relaxing workout.

Day 19: High-Intensity Interval Training (HIIT)

HIIT workouts are intense, but they can be over in a relatively short amount of time. For this workout, choose exercises that use your whole body and alternate between high-intensity and low-intensity movements. For example, you could do 30 seconds of jumping jacks followed by 30 seconds of rest, repeating the pattern for 15 minutes.

Day 20: Active Rest Day

Take a break from structured workouts and focus on being active in other ways. Go for a hike, play a sport, or simply do some light stretching or foam rolling. Your body will thank you for giving it a chance to recover, and you'll come back to your workouts feeling refreshed and ready to tackle the next five days.

Mixing up your workouts is a great way to keep your fitness journey interesting and prevent boredom. By trying different types of exercise, you can challenge your body in new ways and see better results. Remember to listen to your body, rest when needed, and have fun!

Day 21-25: Challenging Your Limits

Days 21 to 25 of a thirty-day fitness challenge can be a critical time in which you challenge your limits and push yourself further. At this point in the challenge, you have built a foundation of strength, endurance, and discipline, and it's time to take things to the next level.

One way to challenge yourself is by increasing the intensity of your workouts. This can mean doing more reps, lifting heavier weights, or doing more challenging exercises. For example, you can add lunges, push-ups, or squats to your routine to target different muscle groups and build overall strength. You can also try interval training, which involves alternating between high-intensity and low-intensity exercises to push your limits and get your heart rate up.

It's crucial to have a strong support system during this time. Surround yourself with people who believe in you and encourage you, and don't be afraid to reach out for help if you need it. Whether it's a workout buddy, a personal trainer, or a support group, having someone to motivate and encourage you can make all the difference.

Day 26-30: Wrapping Up and Celebrating Progress

Day 26: Reflection

As you near the end of your thirty-day fitness challenge, it's important to take a moment to reflect on your progress. Think back to the beginning of the challenge and consider how far you've come. Have you noticed any changes in your physical appearance or overall fitness level? Have you been able to stick to your daily workout routine and maintain healthy eating habits?

Don't allow it to bother you if you have not accomplished all your goals yet. The important thing is that you've tried and have taken steps towards a healthier lifestyle. Pat yourself on the back for your hard work and dedication.

Day 27-28: Intensify Workouts

Now that you're in the homestretch, it's time to push yourself even further. Intensify your workouts by adding more weight or doing more reps. Try a new type of workout that you've been wanting to try, such as a spin class or a yoga session. The goal is to challenge yourself and push your limits.

Day 29: Reward Yourself

Treat yourself to something special to celebrate your progress. This could be a massage, a shopping trip, or a fancy dinner. Choose a reward that you'll enjoy and that motivates you to continue your healthy habits.

Day 30: Celebrate and Plan for the Future

Today is the final day of your thirty-day fitness challenge. Take a moment to celebrate your achievements and give yourself a pat on the back. You've made significant progress in just thirty days, and you should be proud of yourself.

As you wrap up the challenge, think about your next steps. What do you want to focus on in your fitness journey? Do you want to maintain your current level of fitness or push yourself to the next level? Consider setting new goals for yourself and creating a plan to achieve them.

Chapter Eight

Common Challenges and How to Overcome Them

Starting a thirty-day fitness challenge can be exciting, but also a bit intimidating. Even the most motivated and dedicated individuals can struggle with maintaining their fitness routine, especially as the days go by. However, with a bit of preparation and determination, anyone can overcome these common challenges and see significant progress in just one month.

1. Lack of motivation

One of the biggest challenges people face during a thirty-day fitness challenge is a lack of motivation. Always motivate yourself.

2. Time constraints

Try to make exercise a priority in your daily routine by scheduling it in as you would any other appointment.

3. Plateaus and boredom

Try changing up your exercise routine by incorporating new exercises or activities to keep your body challenged.

4. **Lack of support**

To overcome this, consider joining a fitness community or finding an accountability partner who is also committed to their fitness goals.

5. **Injuries and setbacks**

Injuries and setbacks can be a major roadblock during a thirty-day fitness challenge. To prevent injury, make sure to warm up properly before each workout and listen to your body.

Remember to be patient, stay focused, and celebrate your progress along the way.

Conclusion

A thirty-day fitness challenge is a great program for anyone looking to jumpstart a healthy lifestyle. Whether you're a seasoned fitness enthusiast or someone who's just starting out, the structure, accountability, information, community support, and long-term benefits of a fitness challenge can help you achieve long-lasting healthy habits and attain your fitness objectives. So, why not give it a try and see for yourself how a thirty-day challenge can change your life?